Ready, Set, Baby!: Unlocking Secrets to Boost Your Fertility

Angela H. Manuel

Introduction

Parenthood is a fascinating and transformational adventure filled with love, hardships, and unending delight. The road to parenthood is an astonishing adventure that changes lives forever, from the exciting anticipation of pregnancy to the restless nights and the incomparable joy of holding your infant in your arms. Aptly titled, the bundle of joy that enters your life carries with it a tremendous sense of duty, immense happiness, and an emotional rollercoaster.

Early in the pregnancy, the first thrill or shock happens. As a result, you might cease thinking about your pregnancy all the time, and so will your partner. Your companion's exhaustion and pain serve as a daily reminder. The two of you may have different reactions to learning the gender of your child.

Your partner may notice some things before you do because the pregnancy is happening inside of them. One such instance is when you start to concentrate inside and think about your parenting philosophy.

You might not experience it until you feel your unborn child kick. Most likely, your companion started some weeks prior. This mismatch may cause your partner to worry that you don't love your child. Be sympathetic to their concerns.

As you start to think about how you want to raise your child, you'll think about how you were raised. You'll wish to follow in your parents' footsteps in certain ways. There will be things around that you won't. You could even have vowed never to carry out some of these actions. Many expectant parents think it's helpful to talk to their own family. Many people think it's helpful to talk to other expectant parents and new parents.

One difficult issue is when your partner worries about your interest in and acceptance of your child. It's probable that your partner spends some time preparing for the addition of their child to the household.

Making sure your partner will assist:

- Set aside time each week for talking about your pregnancy and the baby.
- Focus on parenting and parenting-related literature.
- Select a name for your child after looking through a name book.
- Say what about your partner you think will make them a great parent, and let them say the same about you.
- Participate in selecting the healthcare provider who will look after your child.
- Consider watching a friend's or relative's kid practice childcare.
- Stop asking out loud what your partner wants. You could ask. Listen to your partner's suggestions.

Try not to worry excessively about your parenting in private. Share your ideas and feelings with your partner about being a parent; they will definitely share your sentiments. Even if you don't feel like you currently have all the answers, discussing the situation with your partner will help them understand that you are taking part in the pregnancy and are anticipating the birth of your child.

What you and your partner should discuss:

- What conclusions may we draw about babies based on our prior encounters?
- How interested are you in learning more about child rearing and parenting?
- How can we ease the stress of the first few weeks following the birth of our child?
- How long do you intend to be away from the office?
- For how long do you want me to be gone?
- What if I'm not particularly good at burping, changing diapers, or rocking our kid to sleep?
- Do you have any suggestions for things I may do to actually assist you right now while I'm pregnant?

- Who should be present when the baby is born?
- Can you help me think of some significant and advantageous things I can begin doing as soon as the child is born?
- Which individuals do we want to be there for us after the birth of our child?

Connecting with your child

To feel closer to your unborn child throughout pregnancy, you can do the following:

- Schedule an ultrasound so you can view your child on the screen.
- Sing and talk to the child you're carrying. If you do this, your infant will recognise your voice. Your infant will turn to face you when they hear you.
- To calm your baby, gently touch your partner's abdomen. You will be able to stroke your baby's foot or hand later on in the pregnancy when your partner's belly swells.

- Write a letter, song, or poem for your child.
- Build or make a present for your child.

•Understanding Fertility

A good way to increase your chances of getting pregnant is Knowing your menstrual cycle. The first phase begins with the first day of your period's bleeding. Your body produces hormones such as follicle-stimulating hormone (FSH) that cause the eggs in your ovaries to expand. Between days 2 and 14, those hormones also aid in the thickening of your uterine lining in preparation for a fertilised egg. This is called the follicular stage.

What Takes Place During Ovulation

The typical menstrual cycle lasts 28-35 days. Ovulation occurs between days 11 and 21 of your cycle. Luteinizing hormone (LH) levels rise, signalling the release of the most mature egg. At the same time, your cervical mucus becomes more slippery to assist sperm in reaching the egg.
It's all about timing.

Women are born with approximately 1 million to 2 million eggs, but only 300 to 400 are released through ovulation during their lifespan. Normally, you only release one every month. The egg passes through one of the two fallopian tubes that connect the ovaries to the uterus. If the conditions are favourable, sperm may fertilise it on its route to the uterus. If the egg is not fertilised within 24 hours of leaving the ovary, it dissolves. Because sperm can live for 3 to 5 days, knowing when you ovulate might help you and your partner plan sex for when you're most likely to conceive.

Keep Track of Your Most Fertile Days

In general, intercourse occurs 1-2 days before ovulation for the best possibility of conception. If you have a 28-day cycle, count back 14 days from the start of your next period. Plan on having sex every other day, say, on days 12 and 14. Because your cycle may be longer or shorter than normal, an internet ovulation calculator or over-the-counter ovulation and fertility kits might assist you in determining the most likely day.

Keep Track of Your Most Fertile Days

In general, intercourse occurs 1-2 days before ovulation for the best possibility of conception. If you have a 28-day cycle, count back 14 days from the start of your next period. Plan on having sex every other day, say, on days 12 and 14. Because your cycle may be longer or shorter than normal, an internet ovulation calculator or over-the-counter ovulation and fertility kits might assist you in determining the most likely day.

Hormone Prediction for Ovulation

An increase in LH causes your ovaries to release an egg. The surge occurs 36 hours before the egg is discharged. Ovulation kits and fertility monitoring kits detect ovulation by measuring LH levels and other hormones. These kits, which employ hormones or are worn as devices, are convenient and highly accurate. You should test 1-2 days before the expected surge to observe the rise in LH.

The Final Stage of Your Monthly Cycle

The hormone progesterone kicks in during the second half of your menstrual cycle to help prepare the lining of your uterus for a fertilised egg. If the egg is not fertilised and does not implant, it disintegrates, progesterone levels fall, and the egg, along with blood and tissues from the uterine lining, is expelled from the body 12 to 16 days later. Menstruation is the name given to this procedure. Normally, it lasts between 3 and 7 days.

Fertility is affected by weight.

If you're overweight or obese, decreasing weight can help you get pregnant. According to one study, women with a higher body mass index (BMI) took twice as long to get pregnant as those with a normal BMI. However, a 5%-10% weight loss can significantly enhance ovulation and pregnancy rates. Obesity can also result in infertility and decreased testosterone levels in men. Significant underweight might also result in infertility.

Your Chances of Conception Are Affected by Your Age

Fertility declines with age, particularly around the mid-30s. It also reduces the likelihood of effective fertility treatments. If you're under 35 and have been trying to conceive for more than 12 months, or over 35 and have been trying for more than 6 months, talk to your doctor.

Fertility is declining in older men as well.

According to studies, sperm count and motility, as well as sexual function, decline as men age. However, there is no age at which a man is considered too old to father a kid. According to one study, men over the age of 45 had a harder time getting a woman pregnant once they began trying. If your partner is older, you should consult your doctor about strategies to improve your odds.

How Can Men Increase Fertility?

•Control your stress.
•Stay away from alcohol and smoke.
•Keep a healthy weight.
•Include zinc (found in meat, whole grains, seafood, and eggs), selenium (found in meat, seafood, mushrooms, cereals, and Brazil nuts), and vitamin E in your diet.
•Keep the testicles cool by avoiding extended, hot baths, hot tubs, and saunas, which can diminish sperm count.

CHAPTER 1

Preparing Your Body

There is a tonne of advice on what pregnant women should and should not do, like limit their intake of caffeine, avoid soft cheeses, and even touch kitty litter.

There is no one optimal moment to begin getting your body and mind ready if you know you want to attempt to get pregnant. In an ideal world, everyone would always prioritise their physical and mental well-being, but in a busy, occasionally stressful world, it's common to put one's own health on the back burner.

If someone is genuinely mindful about getting ready for pregnancy, they should start at least a year or six months in advance.

There are several things you can do to put yourself in the best possible situation to conceive and carry if "Have a baby" is at the top of your to-do list.

1. Compile a family history.
Health problems in your family may develop in you or at least influence how your doctor responds to your inquiries regarding fertility.

Fertility may be impacted by a number of genetic malignancies, including breast, ovarian, cervical, and uterine cancer. It is imperative to let your doctor know if you have a family history with your mother, sister, aunt, or grandmother.

Inform your doctor if you have a family history of any other health disorders that might affect your fertility treatment, such as:

•Diabetes.
•Blood clotting problems.

•Hypertension.

With this knowledge, your doctor will be better equipped to decide whether to do particular screenings, diagnostic tests, or other treatments to help prevent or lessen pregnancy-related issues.

2. Stop using birth control.
Be aware that you may theoretically become pregnant if you quit using birth control, so wait until you're ready.

Contrary to the widespread belief that you should take some time off birth control before trying to conceive, many women can become pregnant pretty rapidly after stopping their contraceptives, provided they don't have an underlying ovulation condition.

3. Commence covering your ovulation.

Your rich window, or the time of the month when you can come pregnant, may not be a commodity you're veritably familiar with yet. Let's talk about ovulation shadowing, which may be done in a number of ways.

• operations for smartphones Some operations use information you supply about your menstrual cycle to read when you'll ovulate.

• Ovulation vaticination strips You may buy these untoward strips to determine if you're ovulating by testing your urine. They're among the most secure at- home styles for determining your rich window.

• rudimentary body temperature charting By tracking your body temperature each morning with a specialised thermometer, you can determine when you've ovulated. It may not be the ideal option while trying to get pregnant, but it can give you further sapience into your cycle.

4. Begin using antenatal supplements

Gestation is the ideal time to establish the habit of taking an antenatal vitamin. Folate, also known as folic acid, is one of their crucial factors since it prevents spina bifida and aids in the normal check of the spinal column in your foetus.

The fresh vitamins and nutrients included in prenatals support and feed both the developing life inside of you as well as you." Nutrients are transferred from the mama to the foetus while a woman is pregnant, therefore it's critical to maintain a steady input of essential nutrients for foetal growth.

5. Learn to manage your stress

Although stress reduction does not directly increase the liability of getting pregnant, there are numerous benefits to it that can enhance your general good and your fertility.

Reducing stress can increase your capability to suppose easily, make opinions with confidence, assess possibilities logically, and have better connections at work, at home, and in other settings.

High quantities of stress can also have an immediate effect on your menstrual cycle, leading you to stop getting your period or indeed have it too constantly, which might vitiate your capability to conceive.

6. Regular exercise

Be active! It's advised to exercise for 30 twinkles each day, at least five days every week.

Exercise helps with stress relief, weight control, and cardiovascular health, all of which are advantages in general but especially when trying to get pregnant.

7. Get to a healthy weight.

As you attempt to get pregnant, talk to your doctor or nutritionist to learn about the right calorie intake, exercise, and other good behaviours. Your weight might affect your ability to get pregnant.

In the case of underweight…

Some underweight people particularly those who suffer from eating disorders like anorexia or bulimia might not ovulate or experience irregular cycles. Even those who are underweight but do not have eating disorders might experience problems with ovulation, cycle control, pregnancy implantation, and preterm birth.

If you're obese…

The health of your eggs and your menstrual cycle are both impacted by obesity. Additionally, those who are overweight are more susceptible to:

•Pregnancy loss and chronic hypertension.

•Diabetes with pregnancy and preeclampsia

I advise obese individuals to attempt to maintain their weight before we put a strategy in place to start losing weight. Start off slowly with five pounds, then ten, then twelve, and we'll go forward from there.

8. Boost your diet.

It's time to change your eating habits if you've been intending to. Consider adopting a diet that leans towards:

- Less consumption of carbohydrates; more consumption of protein and good fats
- a lot of fresh produce.

Typically, a Mediterranean-style diet low in carbohydrates and high in leafy green vegetables is advised. Basically, everything that is vividly coloured in the produce section is likely to be packed with beneficial nutrients.

Several foods should be avoided when you are pregnant as well. To make things simpler for yourself when the time comes, you may consider cutting them out if you presently consume a lot of them before becoming pregnant. Reduce your consumption of predatory fish, such as tuna, which might expose you to higher amounts of heavy metals, including cadmium and mercury.

9.Give up smoking.

Infertility is recognised to be at risk due to smoking. Just one cell layer separates our lung cells from the blood vessels in the lungs, so everything we consume, like cigarettes or marijuana, enters the circulation and travels throughout the body.

Every substance in cigarette smoke accumulates in the body, including the ovaries. Therefore, smoking can have a significant negative effect on ovarian function, egg quality, and egg production. It's preferable to abstain from smoking altogether. To increase your chances of having a healthy pregnancy, try stopping smoking if you currently smoke.

10. Reduce your caffeine intake.

When attempting to conceive, you don't have to give up your morning coffee. However, you might want to reduce your intake if you usually drink a few morning cups. It has been proven that consuming 500 milligrammes or more of caffeine daily, or the equivalent of five or six cups of coffee, might affect fertility and miscarriage.

When you're trying to get pregnant, consider keeping your intake of caffeinated beverages (such as coffee, tea, and soda) to no more than two per day.

11.Discuss your medicine with your doctor.

Numerous drugs might have an influence on your foetus after you get pregnant, as well as on your capacity to conceive.If you're attempting to get pregnant, go through your list of prescription drugs with your doctor and ask whether any of them might affect the pregnancy.

Some typical drugs that could have an impact on foetal development include:

- Methotrexate is a medication for rheumatoid arthritis.
- Isotretinoin is a medication for acne.

- Valproic acid, which is used in the management of seizures,
- Warfarin and other anticoagulant drugs
- ACE inhibitors, which are used to treat various heart problems and reduce blood pressure,
- A few antibiotics, such as tetracycline and doxycycline.
- A number of antidepressants and anxiety drugs, such as paroxetine, lithium, and diazepam.

There is good news before you freak out about discontinuing a prescription that is essential to your personal wellness: in many circumstances, your doctor may point you towards a safer substitution. However, if there isn't an option, your doctor will carefully collaborate with you to explore the dangers of using the medicine while pregnant and decide the best and safest course of action for both you and your foetus.

When to bring up the subject of infertility

Trying to get pregnant while repeatedly finding only one line on pregnancy tests can be upsetting and even devastating. It could be time to consult a doctor if you've been trying for six months to a year without success.

•Nutrition and Diet

Why is the right diet crucial during pregnancy?

One of the finest things you can do when pregnant is to eat properly. As your pregnancy continues, greater demands on your body may be managed with a good diet. The goal is to strike a balance between keeping a healthy weight and consuming enough nutrients to support the growth of your foetus.

The adage "eat for two" is popular when you're expecting, but we now know that eating twice as much food is unhealthy.

Why is nutrition important during pregnancy?

One of the finest things you can do when pregnant is to eat properly. As your pregnancy continues, greater demands on your body may be managed with a good diet. The goal is to strike a balance between keeping a healthy weight and consuming enough nutrients to support the growth of your foetus.

Although the common proverb "eat for two" applies when you're pregnant, we now know that eating twice as much food as usual when pregnant is risky. Instead of "eating for two," try eating twice as healthily.

Starting in the second trimester (and a little more in the third), you require an extra 340 calories per day if you are pregnant with one fetus. That is approximately the number of calories in a glass of skim milk and a half-sandwich.

You should take an additional 600 calories every day if you are pregnant with twins. Eat 900 more calories every day if you are expecting triplets.

Minerals and vitamins are necessary for every bodily process. All the vitamins and minerals you require throughout pregnancy should be given via a nutritious diet and daily prenatal supplement use.

Just one amount of your daily prenatal vitamin should be taken. To determine how many pills make a daily serving, check the bottle. Your obstetrician-gynaecologist (ob-gyn) may suggest it as a separate supplement if they think you require a higher dosage of a vitamin or mineral.

Never take more pregnancy vitamins than what is suggested each day. At larger quantities, several chemicals in multivitamins, such as vitamin A, can result in birth abnormalities.

Folic acid, iron, calcium, vitamin D, choline, omega-3 fatty acids, B vitamins, and vitamin C are important during pregnancy. For the suggested numbers, see the table below.

Important pregnancy vitamins and minerals

Why You Need This Nutrient (Daily Recommended Amount) for Yourself and Your Unborn Child;

(1,300 mg of calcium for those 14 to 18 years old; 1,000 mg for those 19 to 50 years old).

improves bone and tooth strength.

Milk, cheese, yoghurt, sardines, and leafy greens are all good options.

The iron concentration is 27 milligrammes. Assists red blood cells in providing oxygen to the foetus.

Iron-fortified cereals, lean red meat, lean fish, dry beans and peas, and prune juice

220 milligrammes of iodine, necessary for proper brain development.

Dairy products, shellfish, meat, some breads, eggs, and iodized table salt.

It has a weight of 450 grams. Choline, Important for the brain and spinal cord development of your foetus

Other ingredients include dairy, soy, peanuts, beef liver, and others.

•From 14 to 18 years old, vitamin A requirements rise to 770 mcg for individuals in their fifties.

Generates healthy skin and vision.

Aids with bone development.

Carrots, green leafy veggies, and sweet potatoes.

80 milligrammes of vitamin C are advised for people aged 14 to 18; 85 milligrammes are indicated for those aged 19 to 50.

Promotes healthy teeth, gums, and bones.

Cabbage, tomatoes, strawberries, strawberries, strawberries, and more strawberries.

600 international units of vitamin D.

The teeth and bones of your foetus are developing.

Enhances skin and eye health.

Sunshine, fortified milk, and fatty fish like salmon and sardines are all good sources of vitamin D.

Dosage of vitamin B6 (1.9 mg).

Red blood cell production.

Helps in the utilisation of carbohydrates, fat, and protein by the body.

Pig, whole-grain cereals, fruits and vegetables, and gammon, gammon liver, and beef.

Dosage of vitamin B12 (2.6 mg)

Maintaining mental fitness.

Red blood cell production.

Milk, meat, fish, and poultry (vegetarians should supplement their meals with supplements).

The amount of folic acid is 600 mg.

Lowers the chance of congenital abnormalities in the brain and spine.

Helps the infant's and placenta's overall development and growth.

Beans, fortified cereal, bread, pasta, orange juice, peanuts, and leafy green vegetables are all good sources of iron. Take a 400-microgram prenatal vitamin every day as well.

What folic acid does:

Folic acid, often known as folate, is an essential B vitamin for pregnant women. Folic acid supplementation may aid in the prevention of neural tube defects (NTDs), which affect the fetus's brain and spine.

How much folic acid should I take?

When pregnant, you need 600 mcg of folic acid every day. Because it is difficult to receive this much folic acid through diet alone, you should begin taking a daily prenatal vitamin containing at least 400 micrograms of folic acid at least one month before becoming pregnant and for the first 12 weeks of pregnancy.

If you have already had a child with an NTD, you should take a folic acid tablet containing 4 mg of folic acid daily for at least three months prior to becoming pregnant and for the first three months of the pregnancy. If you think you require more than 400 micrograms per day, consult with your OB-GYN.

Why is iron so important for pregnant women?

During pregnancy, your body needs iron to make the extra blood that you and your growing foetus require. While not pregnant, you need 18 milligrammes of iron each day. While pregnant, you need 27 milligrammes per day.

How can I make sure I'm getting enough iron?

In addition to taking an iron-containing prenatal vitamin, you should also take iron-rich foods such as beans, lentils, enriched breakfast cereals, beef, turkey, liver, and prawns. You should also eat foods that help your body acquire iron, such as oranges, grapefruit, strawberries, broccoli, and peppers.

To screen for anaemia during pregnancy, blood tests should be taken. If you have anaemia, your obstetrician may urge you to take extra iron supplements.

What calcium-containing foods are there, and what are they?

Calcium aids in the growth of your unborn child's bones and teeth. Calcium needs for children under the age of 18 are 1,300 mg per day. If you are 19 or older, you need 1,000 mg every day.

Milk and other dairy products, such as yoghurt and cheese, are great calcium sources. If you have trouble digesting dairy products, you can get calcium from alternative sources, such as broccoli, fortified foods (cereals, breads, and beverages), almonds and sesame seeds, and sardines.

What is vitamin D, and what foods contain it?

Vitamin D, in conjunction with calcium, helps in the formation of the foetus's bones and teeth. Furthermore, vitamin D is needed for healthy skin and vision. Whether or not you are pregnant, you need 600 international units of Vitamin D every day.

Fortified milk, morning cereal, fatty fish (such as salmon and mackerel), fish liver oils, and egg yolks are all excellent sources of vitamin D.

How can I determine if I'm consuming enough vitamin D?

Vitamin D intake is often insufficient. A test can be performed to determine your blood level of vitamin D if your OB-GYN suspects that you may have low amounts of the vitamin. You might need to take a vitamin D supplement if it is below average.

What foods contain choline, and what is it?

The growth of your foetus's brain depends on choline. It could also aid in avoiding certain typical birth abnormalities. During pregnancy, experts advise getting 450 mg of choline daily.

Chicken, meat, eggs, milk, soy products, and peanuts are all sources of choline. While the body does create some choline on its own, it is not enough to satisfy your needs during pregnancy. Choline is a nutrient that must be obtained from food because it is rarely present in prenatal supplements.

What exactly are omega-3 fatty acids, and which foods are rich in them?

Many different types of fish naturally contain a kind of fat called omega-3 fatty acids. Omega-3 fatty acids could be crucial for both foetal and postnatal brain development.

Omega-3s are also found in flaxseed, whether it be in its ground or oil form. Broccoli, cantaloupe, kidney beans, spinach, cauliflower, and walnuts are additional foods that contain omega-3s.

How much fish should I consume daily to meet my needs for omega-3 fatty acids?

Eat fish or shellfish twice or three times a week before getting pregnant, during pregnancy, and while nursing. Fish portions are 4 ounces (oz).

What kinds of fish should I stay away from?

Different kinds of fish have different amounts of mercury. Birth abnormalities have been connected to the element mercury. Bigeye tuna, king mackerel, marlin, orange roughy, shark, swordfish, or tilefish should not be consumed. The weekly maximum for white (albacore) tuna is 6 ounces. Additionally, look for warnings concerning fish taken from nearby seas.

What are the B vitamins, and which foods are sources of them?

The B vitamin folic acid, generally referred to as folate, is crucial for pregnant women. Neural tube defects (NTDs), which affect the foetus's brain and spine, may be avoided with folic acid supplementation.

Key nutrients during pregnancy include the B vitamins, which include B1, B2, B6, B9, and B12. These nutrients

• Give you vigour

• Provide energy for the growth of your foetus

• Foster clear vision

• Aid in placing the placenta

The recommended daily intake of B vitamins for pregnant women should be included in your prenatal vitamin. Eating foods strong in B vitamins, such as liver, pig, poultry, bananas, beans, whole-grain cereals, and breads, is also a good idea.

What function does vitamin C serve?

An immune system that is healthy requires vitamin C. It also aids in developing healthy bones and muscles. If you are older than 19, you should consume 80 mg of vitamin C daily when pregnant, and if you are younger, you should consume 85 mg.

You may acquire the recommended daily allowance of vitamin C through citrus fruits and drinks, strawberries, broccoli, tomatoes, and daily prenatal vitamins.

How can I drink enough water while I'm waiting?

Don't limit your drinking to times when you are very thirsty. During pregnancy, aim for 8 to 12 glasses of water each day.

How can I create a healthy eating plan when pregnant?

You can plan nutritious meals using a variety of methods. The American MyPlate food-planning manual is one helpful resource. Agency for Agriculture. You may learn how to make healthy food choices at every meal by visiting the MyPlate website at www.myplate.gov.

The MyPlate website provides a MyPlate Plan that outlines how much food to eat depending on your daily caloric needs. The MyPlate Plan is tailored to your preferences.

•Height
•Weight before pregnancy

•Level of physical activity

You may learn how to choose foods from each food category to acquire the vitamins and minerals you need during pregnancy by using the MyPlate Plan. You may reduce the number of calories from added sugars and saturated fats by using the MyPlate Plan.

Which five food groups are there?

•Grains
•Fruits
•Vegetables
•Protein-rich food
•Dairy products

Describe grains.

Grains include tortillas, bread, pasta, muesli, and cereal. Unprocessed grains are ones that still include the entire grain kernel. Whole grains include oats, barley, quinoa, brown rice, and bulgur, as well as goods manufactured from them. Make half of the grain portions in your meals from whole grains.

What kinds of fruit must I consume?

Fruit is available fresh, canned, frozen, or dried. Fruit juice that is 100 percent fruit juice qualifies as fruit; however, it is recommended to consume the entire fruit rather than juice on a regular basis. When you eat, fill half of your plate with fruit and vegetables.

What kinds of veggies must I consume?

Vegetables can be consumed raw, canned, frozen, dried, or juiced entirely. For salads, use dark leafy greens. When you eat, fill half of your plate with fruit and vegetables.

What foods include protein?

Protein may be found in meat, poultry, fish, beans, peas, eggs, processed soy products, nuts, and seeds. Each day, eat a mix of proteins.

Dairy products are what?

The dairy category includes milk and its byproducts, such as cheese and yoghurt. Any dairy products you consume should be pasteurised. Choose kinds that are fat-free or low-fat (1%).

Why are fats and oils necessary?

Oils and fats are an additional component of a balanced diet. Despite not being a dietary category, they do provide you with vital nutrients. During pregnancy, the fats that you eat give energy and help grow the placenta and numerous foetal organs.

What are healthy sources of oils and fats?

Oils in food are generally derived from plants, such as olive oil, nut oils, and grapeseed oil. They can also be found in specific foods, such as shellfish, avocados, almonds, and olives.

Your diet should mostly consist of plant-based fats and oils. Reduce the consumption of solid fats, such as those obtained from animals. Solid fats can also be found in processed meals.

How much weight should I gain when pregnant?

Before becoming pregnant, your health and body mass index (BMI) will impact how much weight you gain. If you were underweight prior to pregnancy, you should gain more weight than someone who was average weight. If you were obese or overweight before becoming pregnant, you should lose weight. The rate of weight gain varies each trimester.

During your first trimester, the first 12 weeks of pregnancy, you may only gain 1 to 5 pounds, if at all.

If you were at a healthy weight before becoming pregnant, you should gain half to one pound per week in your second and third trimesters.

See the table below for an appropriate weight gain during pregnancy.

Gaining Weight While Pregnant: Prior to pregnancy, BMI Weight Gain Rate* in the Second and Third Trimesters (Pounds Per Week) Total Weight Gain With a Single Foetus (in Pounds) Recommendation Total Weight Gain with Twins (in Pounds) Recommendation.

Underweight, weighing less than 18.5 pounds

18.5-24.9 (normal weight)

(Body Mass Index): 25.0 to 29.9

Obese at 30.0 and above

*A weight gain of 1.1 to 4.4 pounds is assumed throughout the first trimester.

How many additional calories should I eat?

During the first trimester of pregnancy with one foetus, no extra calories are usually required. The following are some examples:

You will require an additional 340 calories per day during the second trimester and roughly 450 calories per day during the third trimester. Have nutrient-dense snacks on hand, such as nuts, yoghurt, and fresh fruit, to receive the extra calories throughout the day.

How might complications during pregnancy be caused by being overweight?

Several pregnancy and delivery issues are linked to being overweight during pregnancy, including:

Blood pressure is high.

- Preeclampsia
- Preterm delivery
- Pregnancy diabetes

Pregnancy-related obesity raises the risk of:

- A foetus that is macroscopically big
- Birth harm
- Caesarean section
- Birth deformities, including NTDs.

•Exercise and Lifestyle

You can increase your fertility (ability to get pregnant) by exercising or being active. Those who routinely engage in moderate exercise become pregnant more quickly than those who don't.

Anything that can help you lose weight is OK; a fitness class in the gym isn't necessary.

• Increase heart rate
• Make breathing easier.
• Give you a warm feeling.

You shouldn't have to stop talking to catch your breath. For instance, brisk walking qualifies as moderate exercise.

Intense exercise may increase your fertility if you have a high BMI and are not getting pregnant as quickly as you had hoped.

Read more if you frequently engage in challenging, rigorous activity.

Being active and exercising for work.

Before and after becoming pregnant, staying active by engaging in regular, moderate exercise will help you have a healthy pregnancy and delivery. According to research, exercising before and throughout the first trimester of pregnancy can lower your chance of developing pregnancy-related issues like gestational diabetes or pre-eclampsia.

Remaining steadfast and prepared for labour.

The body is under stress throughout pregnancy. If you are healthy and strong, you could find it simpler to handle. Additionally, it has been demonstrated that active pregnant women had simpler labours.

Reduce tension and worry.

A baby's birth may be a highly joyous time. Both expectant parents may experience anxiety during this period. You are preparing for a significant shift in your life. Anxiety and sadness are two mental health issues that can be prevalent during pregnancy.

Maintaining an active lifestyle can improve your mood and reduce your vulnerability to stress and sadness.

Advantages for a baby's health

Your child's long-term health will also benefit from continued activity. Children born to active women are more likely to grow up to be active adults. You and your spouse might find it beneficial to consider starting a fitness routine as part of your parent-preparation efforts.

Consider the activities you would like to engage in when you are pregnant and after the birth of your child, and begin planning them now. For instance, it may be taking a stroll around the park or swimming.

You are not required to join pricey gyms or adhere to a tight fitness schedule. It's about putting an emphasis on how to incorporate exercise into daily life.

I should be exercising how much, exactly?

If you've always had a moderate level of activity, for the majority of women, it is safe and beneficial to continue exercising at the same level before (and during) pregnancy if you have always been active.

A tiny percentage of women, including competitive athletes, who work out hard most days of the week may be recommended to reduce their activity to a moderate level if they are having trouble conceiving.

If you haven't been active previously, start increasing it right away. The recommendation is to work up to at least 150 minutes of moderate aerobic exercise per week and strength exercises performed on two or more days of the week that target all the major muscles, or 75 minutes of vigorous exercise per week and strength exercises performed on two or more days of the week that target all the major muscles, or a combination of moderate and vigorous aerobic exercise per week and strength exercises performed on two or more days of the week that target all the major muscles.

Any exercise that causes an increase in heart rate, quicker breathing, or body temperature is considered moderate activity. You shouldn't have to stop talking to catch your breath.

Suitable instances include:

- Swimming
- Slow walking
- Dardening
- Dancing.

Any exercise that causes you to breathe quickly and forcefully qualifies as vigorous exertion. You won't be able to speak for more than a few words without stopping to catch your breath if you're working at this level.

Suitable instances include:

- Running or jogging
- Aerobics
- Tennis singles

Exercises that help build muscles include:

- Heightening objects
- Using resistance bands for exercise
- Sit-ups or push-ups
- Yoga
- Pilates.

Strength training should be done until it becomes difficult for you to continue in order to get the health advantages.

5 suggestions to stay active

1. Don't sit down as much as you can.

Reduce the amount of time you spend sedentary (sitting down). You could try:

- Riding a bike or walking to work
- Getting off a stop sooner or standing when boarding a bus or train
- Visiting a coworker's workstation in person rather than through phone or email
- Creating a phone reminder to stand up frequently

- Choosing the escalator or elevator over the steps

2. Consider using an app like Couch to 5K or Active 10.

Numerous individuals who never imagined they could be active receive assistance from these NHS applications to get started on the path to fitness.

3. When you have a lunch break, go to the park.

if one is available close by. If not, go for a stroll. If at all possible, avoid sitting at your desk at lunch.

4. If it's not too far, walk your other kids to creche, preschool, or toddler group if you have any. An ingenious way to become more active is to turn a daily occurrence into a physical activity. Additionally, it will keep your kids healthy.

5. Install a pedometer app on your phone.

6. They motivate you by showing you how much you are accomplishing by tracking your steps and providing little incentives.

Infertility and exercise

Fitness and a low BMI

Your weight may be too low if your BMI is less than 18.5. There are several causes for underweight people. One explanation may be engaging in too frequent or intense exercise without consuming enough calories to replenish the energy used.

Any exercise that causes you to breathe quickly and forcefully qualifies as vigorous exertion. You won't be able to speak for more than a few words without stopping to catch your breath if you're working at this level.

Fertility issues may result if you lose too much body fat through strenuous exercise, since it may prevent you from ovulating or releasing eggs. A low BMI also carries health hazards for the unborn baby.

Bringing down your level of activity to a moderate level and making sure you eat enough food to replace the energy spent during exercise may assist if you have been trying to conceive and/or do not have regular periods.

Exercise intensity and fertility

The majority of women who are accustomed to strenuous, intensive activity are unaffected by infertility and may maintain their current level of exercise during conception, pregnancy, and beyond.

A few women, such as professional athletes, who regularly engage in strenuous, intensive exercise and have low or healthy BMIs experience infertility. If you don't get regular periods, this is more likely to be the case.

This may be the case because the hormones in your body that control your period might be impacted by the stress that vigorous exercise causes on the body. This may lead to:

- Oligomenorrhea, often known as irregular periods
- Amenorrhoea, or the cessation or absence of periods

Bring down your level of activity to a moderate level and make sure you eat enough to replace the energy consumed during exercise if you exercise vigorously and have been having trouble becoming pregnant or do not have regular periods.

If you've been trying for a year or six months without success, consult your doctor. If you require any tests or treatments, a specialist may be recommended to you.

When should you consult your doctor about fitness and fertility?

If you want to get pregnant but are worried about how exercise will affect your fertility or menstrual cycle, talk to your doctor.

Workout and IVF

One kind of fertility treatment is IVF. In general, people receiving IVF therapy should follow the same exercise recommendations as those who are attempting to conceive naturally.

It has not been demonstrated that moderate physical exercise causes infertility to rise and is safe and healthy. If you exercise vigorously or intensely and are receiving IVF therapy for ovulation issues, your consultant may advise reducing your exercise during treatment to a moderate level.

Men who work out

The link between excessive exercise and male infertility cannot be established with sufficient data. If your spouse is very active and is worried about his or her fertility, he or she could be recommended to exercise less, but other variables are likely to be at play.

Even so, it's crucial that your spouse be active. Overweight people are more likely to be inactive. Being overweight in males might have an impact on the amount and quality of their sperm.

As you are ready to have a child together, you and your spouse might find it beneficial to encourage one another to live healthier lifestyles.

•Managing stress

How to Decrease Stress While Trying to Get Pregnant

One of the most exciting periods in a person's life is when they decide to have a child, but as yet another month goes by with no good outcome, the thrill eventually starts to wane.

Exercise is a simple, healthy approach to reducing stress. You should engage in any physical activity that appeals to you and that you find enjoyable enough to maintain over time. You may like outdoor hobbies, which have the extra benefit of being in the great outdoors, which is a mood enhancer in and of itself, or you may enjoy team sports like basketball or volleyball, or you may prefer solitary pursuits like gardening or bike rides.

Find a conversation partner.
If you need to discuss your problem with an unbiased person who is aware of your struggles, a psychologist, counsellor, or fertility support group might be helpful. A skilled expert can assist you with marital problems, respond to inquiries from family and friends, and control your emotions when other couples conceive while you are unable to.

But be careful not to get mired in them. Talking constantly about your concerns and speculating about potential reasons why they're not occurring might be a trap that is easy to slip into. It loses its usefulness at this point.

Give social media a rest.
According to several studies, the more time spent online, the more nervous and unhappy you may feel. Human nature tends to judge our life

decisions and compare us to others, especially when we're not feeling our best.

feeling too upbeat. Seeing friends online share their family photos and announce their pregnancy can be demoralising for couples who are having trouble becoming pregnant.

Limit your social media usage, especially at night when you ought to be relaxing and calming down from the day.

Study mindfulness and meditation.
Stress can be lessened by living in the now rather than always dwelling on the past or the future. Both mindfulness and meditation are very effective techniques for clearing your mind and preventing the accumulation of unfavorable ideas. It helps you to embrace your emotions rather than suppress them.

To get you started, there are many books, applications, free videos, and other resources online. You could discover that mastering a straightforward practice, like breathing exercises, might significantly improve your situation.

Make time to worry.
'Worry time' is a method that may help you if you struggle to stop intrusive, unpleasant thoughts. Set a time and location where you will sit and think about everything that has tried to get your attention when negative thoughts start to creep in, as opposed to giving in to them.

Psychologists and counsellors frequently employ this technique to help you stop persistently troubling thoughts while allowing you to carry on with your daily activities.

Supplementary treatments.
Numerous alternative therapies, such as hypnosis, reflexology, and acupuncture, can promote relaxation and lower stress levels. You may unwind and divert your attention from

pregnancy and fertility by going to a beauty salon, a massage clinic, or a hair salon.

Perhaps all it takes to make you feel better is the act of talking to someone new about something other than infants.

Laugh whenever you can.
Even if it could be challenging, try to recall your routine before starting a family. Comedy clubs and live performances might help you forget about your worries and be in the moment. And laughing is a tried-and-true, powerful stress reliever.

Enjoy your interests, or discover some new ones.
When we are depressed or going through difficult times, it is easy to forget what makes us happy and to stop taking care of our physical and mental well-being. But life starts to grow when we take a chance or do more of what we like. There are numerous lists of enjoyable things to

do that you can do for free online, but here are 20 suggestions:

• Eat breakfast by yourself, spend time reading the news, and observe people.
• View the dawn
• Attend a concert.
• Put the car in gear and go on a road trip.
• Find a fresh podcast.
• Paint, doodle, or colour
• Take pictures of nature, architecture, or cuisine for an hour.
• Play bowling.
• In the park, read a book.
• Relax in a bubble bath.
• Enrol in a class in an activity you normally wouldn't try.
• View old home films or photographs.
• Go boating or fishing
• Look up at the stars in a dark area.
• Examine landscaping or floristry.
• Arrange a private picnic.
• Visit a restaurant or museum you've never been to.

• Go to a trivia event.

• Participate in karting with friends.

• Visit the landmarks in your own city as a tourist.

CHAPTER 2

Understanding Your Cycle

The hormonal process a woman's body goes through each month to get ready for a potential pregnancy is known as the reproductive or menstrual cycle.

What Is a Typical Menstrual Cycle Length?

The first thing to remember is that, despite the fact that the average menstrual cycle lasts roughly 28 days, every woman's cycle is unique. Even the duration of some women's periods might change from month to month. Your period is termed "normal" if it lasts between 24 and 38 days, with Day 1 marking the beginning of your most recent period and Day 38 marking the beginning of your subsequent one. It's beneficial to monitor your cycle to learn what your typical is, especially after stopping birth control. Although there are many excellent apps that can assist you in understanding your cycle (and even attempt to identify your precise day of ovulation), utilising a conventional calendar also helps.

Male ovulation cycle

On the first day of your menstruation, you can start keeping track of your cycle. The lining of your uterus thickens each month during your cycle to get ready for a prospective pregnancy.

Your progesterone and oestrogen levels start to decline if you are not able to conceive. Your body receives a signal to start menstruating (getting your period) when it is at its lowest point. The uterine lining's blood and tissue start to exit your body during this time period. The typical duration of a period is 4 to 8 days.

During the first few days of your cycle, your body is also capable of performing several other reproductive processes. On your ovaries, follicles have fluid-filled pockets that each contain an egg-start to mature typically throughout Days 1–5. One follicle continues to mature during Days 5-8, while the rest are reabsorbed into the ovary. The amount of oestrogen hormone in your body keeps increasing as this big follicle develops. By Day 8, period bleeding has typically stopped, and these high oestrogen levels have begun to cause the uterine lining to thicken once more. The blood and nutrients in the thickening lining provide the ideal environment for an embryo's nourishment.

Ovulation and the Fertile Window, Days 9-14

The luteinizing hormone (LH) spikes sharply a few days before the big day (Ovulation Day, of course), when oestrogen levels are at an all-time high. The egg is then released from the ovary as a result of the fully-mature follicle bursting (this release normally takes place around Day 14). The best time to try to conceive is during this window of opportunity, called the Fertile Window. The likelihood of becoming pregnant increases if you have intercourse on the day you ovulate, but it's also fairly likely to happen during the three days before. If you have sex before you ovulate, the sperm may still be present and prepared to fertilise the newly released egg because a man's sperm can survive in your reproductive organs for three to five days. There are several techniques you can employ to determine your reproductive window and raise your chances of getting pregnant.

Day 15-24: Implantation and Fertilisation

Progesterone, a hormone released by the ruptured follicle during this period, causes the uterine lining to thicken even more. The egg will be assisted in its descent into the uterus by your fallopian tubes, and if it encounters a sperm and is fertilised, it may eventually cling to the uterine lining. A pregnancy formally starts at this step, which is referred to as implantation.

Day 24-28: Are You Pregnant?

Your hormone levels will decline if the egg is not fertilised, which will cause it to start to break apart. Your period will start as a result, and your cycle will restart on Day 1. Have you heard of PMS (premenstrual syndrome)? It's this significant reduction in hormones that can make you feel cranky and depressed. That is the reason.

Mama, please accept my congratulations if the egg is fertilised and implants in the uterus. You have a baby! Even though a missed period is frequently a reliable early sign of pregnancy, many women use a home pregnancy test to make sure they are indeed pregnant.

It is advised to wait until the first day of your missed period to take a test because hCG levels rise every day of pregnancy. While some tests are more sensitive and claim to be able to identify pregnancy before your missing period, waiting (as difficult as it may be!) will usually result in more accurate findings. A falsely negative test result is more likely the earlier you take the test.

•Identifying Ovulation

When attempting to conceive, it's important to be aware of the symptoms of ovulation, which is the monthly release of a mature egg from one of the ovaries. This is due to the fact that there is just a brief window each month (between 12 and 24 hours) when an egg is viable and you can conceive around the time of ovulation.

Not much of an opening, does it?
So take into account the fact that sperm might survive in the uterus for three to five days. A small amount of sperm may still be present to welcome the egg when it hatches, even if you had intercourse a few days before ovulation.

What signs of ovulation should you therefore watch out for to schedule it perfectly?
Here are the ovulation symptoms you should watch out for if you're trying to get pregnant.
Ovulation indicators
Here are the most typical ovulation signs to look out for: While some women might have few or none of these ovulation symptoms, others might.

1. adjustments to body temperature

Your basal body temperature (BBT) increases a little during ovulation. The two days just before your BBT rises are when you're most fertile. You might be able to more accurately identify your most fertile days by tracking your BBT over a few months with a special thermometer.

However, according to a board-certified reproductive endocrinologist who is also a founding partner and co-medical director of the Colorado Centre for Reproductive Medicine (CCRM) Boston, which opens a new window in Newton, Massachusetts, BBT is not the best way to determine when you're most viable. You might have ovulated a day earlier if BBT rises.

2. modifications in cervical mucus

The cervical mucus thins and becomes more transparent, resembling egg whites in its slippery nature. Your underwear's consistency might have changed.

3. Ovulation discomfort

In your lower abdomen, you can experience a tiny twinge of pain or light cramping (this is referred to as mittelschmerz).

4. Increasing libido

Two to three days before ovulation, your sex desire may become stronger. The most noticeable "male hormone," increased testosterone, is assumed to be the cause of this, which occurs in the ovaries.

5. Vulva alters

The outside of your genitalia, or your labia, could swell.

6. Breast sensitivity

Some women have painful breasts and sore nipples as a result of fluctuating hormone levels.

7. Retention of fluids and bloating

Due to hormonal surges that occur during ovulation, which can cause gas and sluggish digestion, you may suffer bloating and water retention.

8. Mood shifts

Around the time of ovulation, which occurs in the middle of a woman's cycle, some women claim to feel happier and in a good mood.

9. The appetite shifts

You may notice a modest decrease in appetite just before ovulation. It could slightly rise right after ovulation.

10. heightened olfactory awareness

When you are ovulating, which also occurs for some women throughout pregnancy, your sense of smell may get sharper.

Ovulation occurs when?

Ovulation typically happens on day 14 of the typical 28-day cycle, or halfway through your menstrual cycle, when counting from the first day of one period to the first day of the next.

Ovulation often happens 13 to 14 days before your next [anticipated] period, according to a doctor who works with Newton Wellesley Hospital and Beth Israel Deaconess Medical Centre, both in Boston.

As with anything relating to pregnancy, there are many different definitions of normal. Even your own cycle and the timing of ovulation can differ significantly from month to month.

The majority of women have predictable, regular periods, making it easy to anticipate when ovulation will occur.

However, it can be challenging to detect ovulation if your menstruation is irregular, erratic, or comes more frequently than every 40 days.

Try using the ovulation calculator on the What to Expect app to determine your expected fertile window and ovulation date.

What is the duration of ovulation?
12 to 24 hours after ovulation, an egg can be fertilised. The exact time it takes for the egg to be released by the ovary and taken up by the fallopian tube varies, although it typically takes place 12 to 36 hours following an LH surge.

It's recommended to have sex every other day when attempting to get pregnant, starting four to five days before the day of projected ovulation and continuing through the day of ovulation.

Even within this window, some freedom exists. If you have intercourse within 24 hours of the expected ovulation, though your odds may be lower, you can still get pregnant.

Healthy couples who aren't taking birth control typically have a 25 to 30 percent chance of becoming pregnant during each monthly cycle, according to ACOG estimatesOpens a new window. This rate might vary greatly depending on the situation and begins to fall for women in their mid-30s. Of course, increasing the likelihood that a couple may become pregnant by trying to have sex on the day of ovulation.

And keep in mind that all it takes is one sperm to create a child. According to the scientists, this suggests that having intercourse up to five days before and one day after ovulation can result in pregnancy.

Monitor your ovulation
Numerous methods exist for tracking ovulation and determining when you might begin ovulating. Here's how to get ready for ovulation and determine when it will occur:

Keep a menstrual cycle diary.
Keep a monthly cycle calendar for a few months to get a sense of what is typical for you, or use tools like What to Expect Ovulation Calculator to determine the days when you are most likely to ovulate. You should be much more vigilant for other ovulation indicators if your cycles are erratic.

Observe your body.

The B vitamin folic acid, generally referred to as folate, is crucial for pregnant women. Neural tube defects (NTDs), which affect the foetus's brain and spine, may be avoided with folic acid supplementation.

It can be beneficial to keep an eye out for ovulation symptoms in the middle of your cycle. You can have mild cramping, changes in your cervical mucus, breast tenderness, an increase in libido, and mood swings during ovulation.

Does that imply that ovulation can be felt as it occurs?

According to doctors, the answer is indeed yes for some women.

Around the day of or the day after ovulation, some women may experience mild to moderate pelvic pain, cramping, or discomfort in the middle or on one side. This may manifest as a niggling pain or a string of cramps.

This monthly reminder of fertility, known as mittelschmerz (German for "middle pain"), is thought to be caused by the maturation or release of an egg from an ovary. The National Institutes of Health (NIH) Opens a new window estimates that up to 40% of women may be affected. You may be more likely to get the message if you pay close attention.

Keep an eye on your basal body temperature.
That is, your basic body temperature, or BBT. Basal body temperature is the initial reading you obtain in the morning, following at least three to five hours of sleep, and before you get out of bed, speak, or even sit up. It is measured with a specific thermometer.

As your hormone levels fluctuate throughout your cycle, your BBT also changes. Oestrogen predominates in the initial half of your cycle, just before ovulation.

Progesterone levels rise in the period immediately following ovulation, raising your body temperature and preparing your uterus for the eventual implantation of a fertilised egg. According to the NIH, opening a new window means that your temperature will be 12 to 1 degree Fahrenheit higher in the second half of the month than it was in the first.

Confused? The bottom fact is that your basal body temperature will drop to its lowest point just before and during ovulation and then instantly rise by roughly half a degree afterward.

Remember that tracking your BBT for only one month won't help you anticipate when you'll ovulate; it will only provide you with proof of ovulation after it has already taken place. The best way to anticipate ovulation is not to use basal body temperature (BBT). Normal detection of the BBT rise occurs 24 hours after ovulation. There is now an extremely slim probability of becoming pregnant.

However, monitoring BBT over a few months will enable you to identify a pattern in your cycles, allowing you to foretell when your fertile days are and when to go to bed as a result.

The timing of ovulation does vary among women after the drop in temperature, according to studies, and many women find this strategy to be a little disappointing. Kits that predict ovulation are more accurate.

Keep an eye on the discharge
An increase in cervical mucus that is thin and 'watery' is typically the most noticeable indicator of ovulation. The sperm is carried by this cervical mucus, which you'll notice as discharge, to the egg deep within you.

You'll experience a dry phase following the end of your period, so don't anticipate much, if any, cervical mucus. As the cycle continues, you'll notice a rise in mucus production. This mucus is typically white or hazy in appearance and will break apart if you try to stretch it between your fingers.

This mucus increases in quantity three to four days prior to ovulation, but it now has an egg-white-like consistency, is thinner, clearer, and more slippery. How's that for fun in the bathroom? If you try to stretch it between your fingers, you can strain it into a string that is only a few inches long before it snaps. Another indication of approaching ovulation is the presence of this egg white cervical mucus.

Cervical mucus thickens and drastically reduces in volume two to three days following ovulation.

Cervical mucus, when combined with BBT on a chart, can be a very helpful (though rather messy) tool for determining when you're most likely to ovulate, giving you plenty of time to take action.

Some women, especially those who underwent cervical surgery for abnormal PAP smears (such as a LEEP operation), do not generate a lot of cervical mucus.

Get a kit to predict ovulation.
You don't want to play with mucus, do you? You are not required. Many women use ovulation predictor kits, which work by monitoring levels of luteinizing hormone, or LH, the last hormone to surge before ovulation, to forecast the day of ovulation 12 to 24 hours in advance.

Simply pee on a stick, and the indicator will tell you whether or not you are about to ovulate. These kits are more precise than using applications that forecast when you should be ovulating but may not actually be doing so.

If you have regular and predictable periods, ovulation prediction kits are a trustworthy option. It can be challenging to decide when to start tracking if the menstrual interval is irregular or unpredictable. Ovulation predictor kits are unreliable in this situation and may not reliably identify ovulation.

A saliva test, which monitors oestrogen levels in your saliva as ovulation approaches, is a less accurate and infrequently used method. When you're ovulating, the test's eyepiece will show a microscopic pattern in your saliva that resembles the fern plant's leaves or the frost on a window pane. Although not all women have a nice "fern," this reusable test may be less expensive than the kits.

Additionally, there are instruments that can identify the various salts (chloride, sodium, and potassium) that a woman sweats, which alter depending on the day of the month. These tests offer a woman a four-day warning before she may be ovulating, as opposed to the 12- to 36-hour notice that typical ovulation predictors provide. This shift is known as the chloride ion surge, and it occurs even before the oestrogen and the LH surge.

The tests using saliva and chloride ion surge have not been thoroughly investigated and are typically used significantly less frequently.

However, it can't hurt to keep an eye out for these typical ovulation symptoms. Then, do whatever it takes to get you and your spouse in the baby-making mood, such as organise a candlelight dinner, take a warm bath, or go on a romantic weekend vacation.

CHAPTER 3

Boosting Fertility Naturally

Pregnancy plans are frequently put off until later in adulthood. Compared to prior generations, this is different. Despite the fact that women are more fertile naturally in their 20s than in their 30s, children are more frequently born to women between the ages of 30-34. People may believe that it is simple to become pregnant later in life if they see media coverage of female celebrities who do so in their 40s or later. In practice, it could be challenging.

What changes occur to fertility as we age?

As people age, both men and women may experience issues with fertility. All of a woman's eggs are present in her ovaries before birth. Until menopause, a woman's eggs are released throughout her adult life. The eggs eventually expire since they get older with a woman. After the age of 35, it is normally more difficult for women to become pregnant. This is due to the fact that they have fewer and lower-quality eggs. Pregnancy difficulties like miscarriage, gestational diabetes, stillbirth, and genetic abnormalities like Down syndrome are more common in older women.

As a guy ages, his sperm quality may deteriorate. Additionally, miscarriage rates are higher in pregnancies where the dad is over 45. If a woman's spouse is older than 40, it could take her longer to become pregnant.

Women are most fertile when they are younger than 35. The best chance of success in conceiving a child is when you are younger. If a woman is single, she might decide to freeze her eggs. This can be costly and does not ensure a subsequent successful pregnancy.

When should I have sex in order to increase my chances of getting pregnant?

It is advised that a couple engage in sexual activity every two to three days during the fertile phase to improve the likelihood of the sperm and egg forming an embryo. Ovulation time is when a woman is most fertile. Since the egg only survives for 24 hours after being discharged from the fallopian tube, having intercourse before ovulation enhances the likelihood that the egg will be fertilised. The majority of women ovulate 14 days or less before their next period.

A calendar or smartphone app might be useful for keeping track of the menstrual cycle. This can help determine a woman's peak reproductive period. Simple ovulation calendars can be found online. A woman can determine when she is most fertile by observing other physical changes. These include a small increase in body temperature and modifications to vaginal discharge (a fertile woman's cervical mucus is runnier). A woman can use ovulation kits to determine her optimal reproductive window. You can purchase ovulation kits at a pharmacy or online. To measure hormone levels, they can test the urine or the saliva. This displays the likely times for ovulation. Kits for ovulation might be pricey.

What more can I do to increase the likelihood that I will get pregnant?
controlling your weight
Fertility can be impacted by being overweight or underweight. Obese or underweight women are likely not to ovulate on a regular basis. Pregnancy problems like high blood pressure and gestational diabetes are more likely to occur in overweight women. A woman can do the following things to boost her chances of becoming pregnant:

•Eat a nutritious, balanced diet and exercise moderately on a regular basis, as recommended by your doctor.

•A guy can do the following things to boost his chances of getting pregnant:
• Aim for a healthy weight; if you're unsure of the range that is healthy for your height, check with your doctor or nurse. • Eat a healthy, balanced diet.

Smoking

Smoking tobacco (including passive smoking) can lower fertility in both men and women. Sperm production can be potentially impacted by cannabis smoking. Men who smoke are more likely to experience erectile dysfunction, have less sperm, and have lower-quality sperm.
Smoking can: • affect the egg's journey to the uterus in females;
Interrupted hormones have an impact on the placenta's blood vessels, which can influence the growth of the baby.
The odds of miscarriage or stillbirth rising
greater likelihood of childhood asthma
Men and women who smoke should quit if they want to have more children.
drug and alcohol abuse

Australian rules advise against women using alcohol when trying to conceive. Both male and female fertility can be lowered by alcohol. It can lengthen the gestational period,
decrease the calibre of a man's sperm while increasing the calibre of a woman's eggs
Cannabis, ecstasy, cocaine, and heroin can all hinder fertility. Your chances of becoming pregnant will increase if you stop using drugs.

When should I seek assistance?
The majority of healthy couples will conceive within a year of trying. Visit a Family Planning NSW facility or your GP to discuss your options if you are:

If you are under 35 and have tried for one year without success, or if you are over 35 and have tried for six months without success,
It's crucial to speak with your doctor right away if you suspect that you may be experiencing fertility problems.

•Nutritional supplements

Prenatal vitamins should be taken before becoming pregnant, not only after learning you are expecting. There are many other supplements than prenatal vitamins that could boost your fertility and aid in conception. However, since it could take a few months to experience all of the benefits of supplements, it is recommended to begin taking them a few months or more before conception. There are so many supplements on the market. But to make things easy, here are the top six items that will improve your fertility and raise your chances of getting pregnant.

CoEnzyme Q10, often known as Coq10, is a type of natural antioxidant. It is required for the fundamental operations of cells and serves as the mitochondria's fuel supply. Our advice is to take 200–400 mg if you're under 37 years old and 400–600 mg if you're over 37.

D3 vitamin

Studies have it that women still had inadequate levels of vitamin D even after taking a prenatal supplement. A prenatal pill most times doesn't have enough vitamin D added, therefore it's crucial to double verify. Schizophrenia, diabetes, and skeletal conditions have all been linked to low vitamin D levels in children. Diabetes, dementia, autoimmune diseases, and depression can all be prevented with enough vitamin D intake. Take between 2,000 or 3,000 IU daily, as advised.

Folic acid: Preserves the development of the baby's neural tube. According to one study, women who consumed at least 700 micrograms (mcg) of folic acid daily were 40–50% less likely to experience ovulatory infertility than those who consumed less than 300 [1]. Our advice is to consume 400 mcg everyday or more. Selenium: As an antioxidant, selenium shields cells from harm. According to preliminary research, women who use this supplement may be able to avoid miscarriages. It is advised for men to guarantee sperm viability. Take 200 mg every day, as per our advice.

Vitamin E is a natural antioxidant and aids in boosting fertility. Our advice is to consume 500–800 IU.

•Herbal Support

If you're interested in using herbal support, you can increase fertility by taking adaptogens like Ashwagandha or Vitex (chasteberry). Before using herbs as a supplement, do your homework. For instance, ashwagandha may cause adverse effects such as headaches or stomach problems. We advise you to consult your physician or dietitian before taking an herbal supplement.

Additional fertility-boosting supplements:
These are the top six supplements we found to increase fertility. But you should also take into account the advantages of the following:
Omega-3 fatty acids, iron, zinc, vitamins B6 and B12, vitamin C, N-acetyl cysteine (NAC), L-arginine, and acetyl L-carnitine.
To improve your health and fertility, a naturopathic doctor can help you manage nutritional and lifestyle modifications.

CHAPTER 4

Emotional and Psychological Well-Being

You hold your breath each time you check the pregnancy test. Your pulse quickens. Will you be welcomed with happiness or dismay? And will your dismay send you into melancholy if the test results are negative?

Couples and individuals may experience a wide range of emotions and difficulties as a result of infertility. It is something that significantly affects how you travel.

The psychological implications of infertility and mental health, the value of seeking help, and the importance of self-care will therefore be examined in greater detail.

Understanding the Relationship Between Mental Health and Infertility

Women who experience infertility frequently experience a wide range of complex emotions that have an emotional and psychological impact. It's common to feel various emotions, including:

Grief, depression, anxiety, hopelessness, and a great deal of stress

Those struggling with infertility and mental health may experience societal and cultural demands to start a family, which only serves to exacerbate matters further. Even just being around young children can be quite painful emotionally.

The Importance of a Support System

You need a support system to get through the arduous and devastating battle of infertility. Important individuals in your support network could be:

- Your health care team at Chapel Hill OBGYN: friends, loved ones, family, a therapist or professional counsellor, or a member of the clergy support groups
- Reaching out to an understanding friend, loved one, or family member might help

you feel better mentally because infertility can be an isolated situation.

- Sharing your feelings with people who genuinely care about you can help them understand and validate your feelings. Be open and transparent about your infertility and mental health challenges. This significantly reduces feelings of loneliness and self-doubt.

Additional practical support is required.Even though we have emphasised the advantages of emotional assistance, there is still a need for practical support. Treatments and checkups for infertility can be mentally and physically draining.

Never hesitate to enlist the assistance of your loved ones. They can help in the following ways:

•Helping with domestic duties, running errands, and transporting you to doctor's visits preparing meals. You'll have the time and room to devote to your health as a result of this.

•Online support groups for mental health and infertility. Online infertility support communities also exist, offering a secure setting for people to interact with one another, exchange stories, and find comfort in a group of people going through comparable challenges.

These can offer a secure setting for discussing infertility and mental health.

Suggestions for Self-Care When Dealing with Infertility and Mental Health

While coping with the difficulties of infertility, putting mental health first is crucial. Self-care practices can boost mental health in general and give one a sense of empowerment. We urge you to think about including the following in your usual schedule:

Meditation and mindfulness

These procedures employ methods that:

•Deep relaxation, nonjudgmental observation of thoughts and emotions, and developing present-moment awareness

•A higher ability to deal with the difficulties of infertility is also fostered by mindfulness and meditation, which strengthen emotional resilience.

•You can develop a more optimistic mentality, enhanced general wellbeing, and better acceptance on your path to motherhood by centering yourself in the present and engaging in self-compassion exercises.

Take care of yourself.

A crucial part of the path is developing self-compassion and setting reasonable goals. Permit yourself to cry and to be angry. Try not to suppress your emotions. Give your spouse or partner space to experience and deal with you in different ways.

Honestly and openly communicate with your partner.

When dealing with the difficulties of infertility, it is essential to have an open and honest dialogue with your partner. You provide a secure environment for comprehension and support by sharing your ideas, anxieties, and feelings.

Expressing your needs to one another; allowing space for a deeper connection and empathy; actively listening to your partner's perspective; acknowledging that your partner may be feeling different emotions than you do; talking openly about your experiences; allowing time for each other to express concerns;

Together, you may make decisions and seek the right support as you navigate the ups and downs of the infertility journey.

Engage in pleasurable activities.

Sometimes engaging in enjoyable activities might help lower stress. When suffering from infertility and mental health, it's important to do things you enjoy.

Making time for activities that improve your emotions and make you happy is important because infertility can be emotionally taxing. You might think about learning a new pastime, being outside in nature, listening to music or playing an instrument, scheduling time for an old interest, etc. going for a walk or enrolling in a programme for exercise

Think about the advantages of expert therapy or counselling.

Keep in mind that there are therapists who focus on supporting those who are experiencing infertility. Your concerns, struggles, and anxieties can be discussed in a secure setting with a therapist.

Review your social skills and relationship management.

Keep in mind that you might need to explain your needs to others. What someone believes will assist often does not.

Say so if you need to skip the family gathering with the five under-two nieces and nephews. Asking will increase your likelihood of receiving what you want, whether you desire a hug, a massage, some alone time, or nothing more than to be heard.

It's crucial to talk to loved ones about infertility so they can support you and help you comprehend the sensitive issues involved.

Keep in mind that handling social settings, especially pregnancy announcements, can be emotionally difficult. If necessary, reach out to your support network or therapist.

•Support Networks

Being infertile can make you feel alone and alienated, and family and friends frequently struggle to fully comprehend what you're going through. There are infertility support groups created with you in mind, whether you're looking for guidance about your fertility issues or you need support when you begin in vitro fertilisation (IVF) or another treatment strategy. Look to these organisations for empathy and support throughout your fertility journey.

Why is encouragement throughout fertility treatments so crucial?

In addition to being physically taxing, fertility treatments can be emotionally draining for both you and your partner.

It can be reassuring to realise you're not alone by joining a support group, whether it be in person or online. There are groups for both sexes that include participants, which will make you feel at ease and understood.

How to locate regional support groups for infertility

Our employees take pleasure in always being available to meet our patients' urgent requirements at The Fertility Institute of New Orleans. In order to help you navigate fertility issues, we are pleased to direct you to local resources or our own support groups that meet in-clinic. For more information, only ask your doctor at your subsequent appointment. We're prepared to assist.

If you live outside of the New Orleans region, RESOLVE is a fantastic resource for those who are having trouble conceiving a child. You can get in touch with resources in your neighbourhood with the aid of this nonprofit organisation.

Online support groups for infertility

Because infertility issues are personal, joining an online support group might be beneficial. If you don't feel comfortable sharing your personal journey in person with your neighbours, an online community gives you the option to do so while maintaining your anonymity and receiving written support whenever you need it.

Here are four online infertility support groups that provide supervised and secure help if you're interested in making a connection with a group.

Facebook page for the IVF Support Group

The IVF Support Group is a sizable Facebook community for people who have undergone or are undergoing IVF, with close to 27,000 members.

This is a space for closed-door group storytelling and suggestion-sharing. Only group members have access to shared content. If discussions get sour or tense, moderators can intervene.

•Mind-body Connection

Teaching mind-body tools to women going through infertility has been proven to more than double pregnancy and IVF success rates. This amazing statistic has been repeated across multiple research studies over the last few decades and shows an exciting way that women can boost their natural fertility and improve their fertility journeys.

What is the mind-body connection?

The mind-body connection is an increasingly popular approach that sees our mind and body working together for optimal health. Typically, we view our bodies as separate entities and our health as having nothing to do with our thoughts, emotions, and stress levels.

We all know where we hold stress in our bodies and also how negative emotions can manifest themselves in symptoms in the body. We also know that stress can cause headaches, tense muscles, high blood pressure as well as digestive issues. There's a whole range of ways our minds can affect the functioning of our bodies.

What does this mean for fertility?

The emotional side of fertility is huge. Research shows that it has as been compared to the same levels of stress and despair as those diagnosed with a terminal illness!

Studies show women suffering from stress, anxiety, or depression are half as likely to conceive as those who aren't. This is mainly to do with the intricate balance of hormones in our bodies, and with regards to stress, the hormones are regulated from the same place as our reproductive hormones, so they can directly impact each other.

Now, that doesn't mean that people with high stress levels can't get pregnant, and if you relax, you will definitely get pregnant. It just means that for the majority of us, the mind plays some role in the functioning of our bodies, so if we can work to get the mind healthy, this has an effect on the body (and a happier, healthier you too!).

Many studies have shown that when stress is reduced or negative emotions are changed to be more positive, the chances of conception are much higher. The chances of conceiving naturally are also higher. One study from Harvard University showed 55% of women getting pregnant following a mind-body programme, versus 20% who didn't, and 76% of them got pregnant naturally within 12 months.

CHAPTER 5

Partner's Role

Pregnancy is frequently viewed as the responsibility of the woman carrying the child, who must time her cycle, make healthy decisions, take vitamins, etc.

Throughout the process of trying to get pregnant, there are many things your spouse can do to support, encourage, and increase your chances of getting pregnant.

Ensure the health of their reproductive system.

Everyone should minimise unhealthy choices when trying to get pregnant, not just you. Your male spouse can take a variety of actions to improve the health of his sperm, such as:

1. Limiting alcohol consumption: Heavy drinking can lower testosterone production and have an impact on fertility.

2. Giving up drugs and/or smoking: Men who smoke or use drugs are more likely to have low sperm counts and/or slowed sperm motility. Additionally, ladies, you must absolutely avoid secondhand smoke.

3. Getting to a healthy weight: Research indicates that a higher BMI may be associated with sperm that are less active and less countable. Additionally, you are more likely to do so if your partner maintains a healthy diet and exercises regularly.

4. Reducing stress: Stress-related behaviours (such as binge drinking and poor sleep)

might interfere with sperm quality and reduce your chances of getting pregnant.

5. encountering their provider: Making an appointment with their doctor can be helpful in determining any medical history or other circumstances that may have an influence on fertility, including prescription drugs that may have some impact on sperm health.

6. Avoiding hotter surroundings: Contrary to popular belief, hot environments like saunas, steam rooms, and hot tubs can cause a man's testicles to heat up excessively, killing sperm and reducing the number. Request that he refrain from using the sauna while you are trying to conceive.

STI detection and treatment

Infertility can be brought on by sexually transmitted diseases like gonorrhoea and chlamydia in both men and women. If you have a male partner, you can get them tested (and, if necessary, treated) to ensure that their sperm is viable and to prevent them from passing an STI to you. Up to 40% of women with these infections may develop pelvic inflammatory disease (also known as PID) if left untreated. PID has the potential to induce fatal tubal (or ectopic) pregnancies as well as infertility.

Be a reliable teammate.

It's essential that both spouses are fully dedicated to trying for a child and that you are both on the same page about your decision to become pregnant. Supportive relationships improve the likelihood that the expectant mother will receive quality prenatal care and that both partners will refrain from dangerous habits (such as smoking, drinking, or using drugs).

It's critical that your partner conduct some research as well, even while you may be reading endless articles, using apps, and brushing up on the details of how a baby is created. When your spouse is familiar with the specifics and jargon of trying to get pregnant, it can make you feel tremendously supported.

Communicating with Your Partner.
All partners involved experience psychological and emotional stress due to infertility. Unfortunately, this stress can show up in ways that harm a relationship. Every connection is built on communication. When faced with difficulties related to infertility, it can be challenging to communicate about feelings and frustrations, yet maintaining solid communication can enhance relationships. We're offering our top infertility communication advice for couples struggling to conceive to help you get through these trying times.

Talk about it.

Talking it out is one of the greatest infertile communication ideas because communication is essential. Even though it might seem simple, taking the time to describe how you're feeling and how these emotions affect your behaviour and reactions can be quite beneficial.

Your partner might find what you find reassuring and your method of handling the circumstances strange or perplexing. To help your spouse better understand what you need, talk about how you're feeling and what supports you. Making time to listen to your partner will help you understand how they handle things and how they are feeling. The greatest strategy to avoid more stressful situations is to give yourself enough time to accurately express your thoughts and feelings. No one likes to feel as though they have to guess or read minds.

Limit Yourself.
Even though communication is crucial, it can be annoying when a conversation seems to go around in circles. Allocate time for talking about

any infertility-related frustrations or concerns, but be strict with yourself. Allow time for both parties to express their feelings, but avoid lingering on the subject.

Make sure you reserve space for talking about the other elements of your life because stressful events might make you feel like you are carrying a massive, all-encompassing weight on your shoulders.

Share obligations.
When thinking about IVF therapy, there are other considerations besides the emotional burden. If you and your spouse decide to seek treatment, be sure to assign different people responsibility for scheduling appointments, paying bills, handling insurance, etc.

Timing is an excellent way to divide things out so that one person handles scheduling, communicating, and conducting research for the appointment. Any bills, insurance claims, or other issues that arise after the appointment are handled by the other party.

Look for assistance outside the relationship.
There is nothing wrong with requesting more assistance. It puts a lot of pressure on your partner, who is only human, to be your main source of support.

To maintain room for fun and enjoyment in your relationship, find a safe place to express how you feel. This could be with a friend, a member of your family, a qualified professional, or even an internet forum.

Establish Limits.
Before sharing any sensitive information, talk limits with your partner before calling a friend or member of your family. Establish clear boundaries for how much sharing you and your spouse are willing to do, and then abide by them.

Helping one another.

The idea that infertility only affects women is a widespread one. That is false, though, as infertility affects both men and women equally. According to the National Institute of Child Health and Human Development,

In one-third of infertile couples, the male partner is at fault.

One-third of the issues are related to women, and the other one-third are due to issues that are either difficult to pinpoint or affect both men and women.

It's important to accompany your spouse on their journey, even if you don't fully get what he or she is experiencing. We at Carolina Fertility Institute are aware of the difficulties infertility causes. Here are some suggestions for helping your partner cope with infertility.

Plan ahead.
The uncertainty that precedes any infertility journey might be lessened with a plan. A

treatment plan for infertility may contain the procedures you want to pursue, a schedule, and a budget.

As soon as you have a strategy in place, occasionally check in with your spouse to make sure you both understand your treatment options and the recommended course of action. And it's always a good idea to go with your spouse to their doctor's appointments if they're okay with it.

Look for distractions.
Finding distractions that can temporarily remove your thoughts from your concerns is a terrific method to connect with your partner, even though it is not advised to do so. Prior to your infertility issues, try partaking in your favourite pastimes. Dinner and a movie, giving back to the community, seeing a performance, or even taking a trip are all great date ideas!

Attend a counselling or support group session.
If it's difficult for you to draw emotional conclusions in private, joining a support group or going to counselling with your partner are fantastic options for talking things out.

You can have access to a qualified specialist who can provide you with advice on how to communicate and support one another through fertility counselling. Additionally, being around people going through comparable difficulties in infertility support groups might help you feel less alone.

Let your emotions go wild.
In these trying times, sticking together can make your relationship stronger than ever. Being present physically and emotionally and allowing whatever emotions, sadness, angst, and frustration come forth is a terrific method to ensure that feelings don't get trapped up. Suppressing feelings can put physical pressure on the body and cause tension, which does little

to help the predicament you and your spouse are in.

Additionally, remember that your sentiments are legitimate while allowing your partner to experience all of their appropriate emotions.

Be persistent.
The most important method to support your partner during their infertility is to be patient. Keep in mind that criticising your partner won't help the situation; instead, it will make it worse. Recognise that you and your spouse may use various coping mechanisms, and practise patience while they separate their feelings without attempting to solve them right away. Reiterate to your mate that you love them and are travelling together in this life.

CONCLUSION

Your Fertility Journey Ahead

Even though many things seem to be beyond your control at the moment, there are still many aspects of this process that you can manage. Therefore, even if you might still wish you had more control over all the puzzle parts, these ten items are equally crucial and help to raise your odds of having the adorable baby you've always wanted.

Did you realise? According to organisational psychologist Loran Nordgren's research, concentrating on intangible barriers (removal of emotional friction) can be more beneficial than making more headway towards your objective. On the Hidden Brain podcast, Nordgren talked about how putting the emphasis on removing barriers might help you face and overcome the apparently insurmountable issues in life. Let's apply this idea to your quest for fertility and concentrate on certain roadblocks you can overcome:

Seek Assistance

Speak to a counsellor who specialises in fertility for a fantastic method to achieve this. Never visited a therapist or counsellor before? Do you doubt their ability to assist you? Make an appointment and try to show up just once.

Decide if it's right for you after experiencing it for yourself.

Request Support

You can ask for assistance without even revealing that you are undergoing fertility issues or treatments. Saying, "I'm struggling with something that I'm not ready to talk about, but I could use some distraction or support," is sufficient.

Consult with people you trust, and consider your response if someone approaches you for assistance. Allow others to assist you, as you would be more than pleased to do so for them!

Here are some such requests you could make:

•A discussion over coffee or tea

•To take a stroll together.

•If you don't feel like cooking, get some assistance.

•To see a humorous movie with them

•In order to remove your "I'm fine!" mask, which is so draining to wear, just telling folks that you're having a hard time may be such a relief.

Take care of yourself.

Make sure you're getting enough rest, food, and self-care whenever you can.

Everyone's definition of self-care is unique, but the most important thing is to give your physical and emotional health the highest priority possible. To do more of the activities that make you feel most like yourself, you might even assign some responsibilities or chores to other people.

Establish Limits.

Setting boundaries for how much information you're willing to share about your reproductive journey is acceptable. Decide what you want to say and what you don't want to say if you want to let people know that you are suffering from anything significant. Even better, create a script and perform it!

Here's an illustration: I'm not feeling well right now, but I'm not ready to discuss it. Instead, I would really like to chat about (insert favourite book, TV show, event, etc.).

Have a few responses prepared for when someone inquires about your family-building intentions; choose the ones that feel most appropriate to you. It's acceptable to use polite comments or even to be a little snarky if that suits your personality.

•"I'll let you know as soon as there is anything about a baby to announce.

•I truly want to know how things are going for you and your family.

"I'm not interested in discussing about me or us bearing a child."

Conduct a private check-in.

Think to yourself, "How am I right now?" When you begin to feel your anxiety rising, take a deep breath. Keep an appreciation diary. Increase your daily meditation time by 5–10 minutes.

There are many methods to check in with yourself, but the most crucial aspect of this is that you're giving yourself space for introspection and acknowledging your emotions.

Go for a break.

Do you believe that you must continue trying, cycle after cycle? Are you certain that taking this action is the right move for you? Do not be reluctant to discuss the possibility of taking a brief (or extended) sabbatical with your doctor.

Even if it seems contradictory, many patients discover that taking a break can greatly reduce pressure, despite the fact that the urge to have a baby is all-consuming. Once you return to treatment, you will be revitalised and full of newfound optimism and vigour.

Take a broad perspective.

My favourite three-letter word is "yet."

It goes without saying that growing your family has already taken longer than you'd like. But it simply hasn't taken place yet.

When you pan out and look at the big image, it appears like that. It can be reassuring to know what comes next in your fertility treatment plan when you change your outlook.

Recognise your treatment strategy.

Review all the information and resources you have received.

Have inquiries? Before you are in the middle of therapy, ask your care team. This will aid in putting some worries or uncertainty to rest. Maintaining a running list of questions for your doctor can also be quite beneficial.

Join a support group to learn from others' experiences and get a sense of what to expect from the process. Investigate pertinent, trustworthy research from institutions like the American Society for Reproductive Medicine (ASRM), but avoid Dr. Google and anxiety-inducing internet "experts."

Establish connections with your care team.

Maintain regular contact with your fertility treatment team and your patient navigator. Inform them of your current situation and any worries you may have. When they are aware of what is happening, they can take better care of you.

Regular communication can also avoid misunderstandings and lay the groundwork for a solid foundation that will serve you well on your trip.

Prioritise open communication.

Don't attempt this alone, if at all feasible. There's a lot to figure out!

Make sure you talk about your feelings with your spouse, if you have one, and inquire about theirs as well. You might also want to schedule a time when you don't discuss any aspect of fertility treatment. If you don't have a partner, think about confiding in other reliable acquaintances or members of your family.